DIABETES DIET RECIPES FOR BEGINNERS

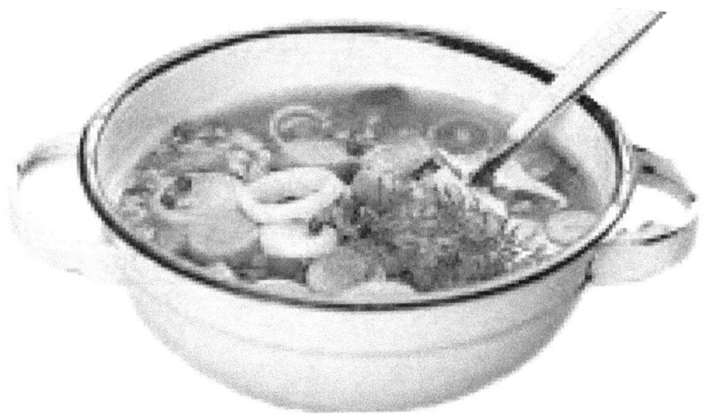

A Healthy Eating Habits for Types 1 and Type 2 Diabetics

Isabelle Hartley

OTHER BOOKS BY THIS AUTHOR

1. RECIPES FOR LOW BLOOD CHOLESTEROL
2. ATKINS DIET RECIPES COOKBOOK
3. CARDIAC DISEASE DIET COOKBOOK
4. CELIAC DISEASE RECIPES COOKBOOK
5. JUICING RECIPES FOR CANCER

TABLE OF CONTENTS

Introduction

"Diabetes Diet Recipes for Beginners" is a comprehensive guide designed to tackle the challenges posed by diabetes, a chronic illness affecting countless lives. Diabetes, with its two primary forms, Type 1 and Type 2, is a pervasive health concern, characterized by the body's inability to regulate blood sugar effectively. The book emphasizes the pivotal role of a healthy, balanced diet in managing diabetes. It serves as the cornerstone of well-being, offering an accessible understanding of diabetes, its variants, and the physiological aspects. Notably, the text explores the role of carbohydrates in regulating blood sugar levels, introducing strategies to make informed dietary decisions and the significance of the glycemic index. Beyond theory, it features an extensive collection of mouthwatering recipes curated for diabetics, dispelling the misconception that such diets are bland. The diversity spans various cuisines, catering to different tastes. The book not only presents delicious recipes but also offers practical advice on portion control, meal planning, and the importance of balanced nutrition. It highlights the value of monitoring blood sugar levels and emphasizes the holistic approach to well-being through exercise and mindful eating. "Diabetes Diet Recipes for Beginners" recognizes the individuality of each person's diabetes journey and encourages personalization and empowerment. Ultimately, it empowers readers to make health-conscious choices, fostering vitality and well-being. This book is more than a cookbook; it is a guide to a healthier, happier future, starting in the kitchen, with support every step of the way.

Samuel's story is a testament to the transformative power of a well-managed diet in the face of diabetes. Samuel, despite having lived a long and fulfilling life, found himself burdened by the unwelcome companion of diabetes as the years passed. His daily routine was marred by doctor's appointments, insulin injections, and a stringent medication regimen, leading to exhaustion from the ceaseless struggle to control his blood sugar levels.

One fateful day, while reflecting in his garden, Samuel resolved to seek a better way to manage his condition. He embarked on a journey of research, delving into the intricacies of diabetes, its root causes, and potential dietary solutions. Through books, online resources, and conversations with healthcare experts, he began to recognize that the key to effectively managing his diabetes lay in the food he consumed.

Samuel's newfound determination prompted a radical transformation in his diet. He bid farewell to sugary snacks, refined carbohydrates, and processed foods, opting instead for a diet rich in whole grains, lean proteins, fresh vegetables, and fruits. His meals were meticulously balanced, and he maintained rigorous monitoring of his blood sugar levels.

Initially met with skepticism from the villagers, who were accustomed to his struggles, Samuel remained steadfast in his commitment to healthier choices. He incorporated regular, brisk walks into his daily routine, tended to his garden, and even took on the role of educating the village's children about the virtues of healthy eating.

Months passed, and something remarkable unfolded. Samuel's blood sugar levels began to stabilize, leading to a decreased dependence on insulin and fewer visits to the doctor. Word of the elderly man who had harnessed the power of diet to conquer diabetes spread throughout the village. Inspired by Samuel's journey, the local grocer began stocking healthier options, and the bakery introduced whole grain bread.

Over the years, Samuel, now in his late 80s, achieved a remarkable reversal of his diabetes. He no longer required insulin or medication, and his vitality surpassed that of his younger years. Samuel's inspiring tale of triumph over diabetes served as a beacon of hope, not only within his village but also resonated with people far and wide.

The story of this elderly man, who had grappled with a debilitating condition, is a living testament to the potential of making the right choices in life. Samuel's unwavering commitment to his health not only prolonged his life but also instilled a newfound perspective on well-being within the entire village. In the serene, sun-dappled village, Samuel's narrative emerged as a powerful symbol of hope and a testament to the life-altering impact of making informed, health-conscious choices.

CHAPTER 1:

Diabetes is a complex metabolic disorder that affects millions of people worldwide. It's a chronic condition that impairs the body's ability to regulate blood sugar levels. Understanding diabetes, its various types, causes, and symptoms is essential for effective management and prevention. In this comprehensive essay, we will delve into the world of diabetes.

Types of Diabetes

There are primarily three types of diabetes: Type 1, Type 2, and gestational diabetes.

1. Type 1 Diabetes:

- Cause: Type 1 diabetes is an autoimmune disorder in which the body's immune system mistakenly attacks and destroys the insulin-producing beta cells in the pancreas. The exact cause is not well understood, but it is believed to involve genetic and environmental factors.

- Symptoms: The onset of Type 1 diabetes is often sudden and occurs in childhood or adolescence. Common symptoms include excessive thirst, frequent urination, unexplained weight loss, extreme hunger, fatigue, and blurred vision.

- Treatment: People with Type 1 diabetes require lifelong insulin therapy, either through injections or an insulin pump, to replace the lost insulin.

2. Type 2 Diabetes:

- Cause: Type 2 diabetes is primarily linked to lifestyle factors, genetics, and insulin resistance. It often develops in adulthood, but the rising prevalence among children and adolescents is a growing concern due to poor dietary choices and sedentary lifestyles.

- Symptoms: The onset of Type 2 diabetes is gradual, and symptoms may not be as noticeable initially. They include increased thirst, frequent urination, fatigue, slow wound healing, and blurred vision.

- Treatment: Lifestyle changes like a healthy diet and regular exercise are crucial in managing Type 2 diabetes. Some individuals may require oral medications or insulin injections in addition to lifestyle modifications.

3. Gestational Diabetes:

- Cause: Gestational diabetes occurs during pregnancy when the body cannot produce enough insulin to meet increased needs. The exact cause is unclear, but hormones produced during pregnancy can lead to insulin resistance.

- Symptoms: Most women with gestational diabetes do not exhibit noticeable symptoms. However, it can lead to complications for both the mother and the baby if not managed.

- Treatment: Managing gestational diabetes typically involves dietary changes and monitoring blood sugar levels. Insulin or other medications may be necessary in some cases.

Common Causes of Diabetes

- Genetics: A family history of diabetes increases the risk of developing the condition. Certain genetic factors can make individuals more susceptible to Type 1 and Type 2 diabetes.

- Insulin Resistance: In Type 2 diabetes, the body's cells become resistant to the effects of insulin. This means the body needs more insulin to maintain normal blood sugar levels. The exact cause of insulin resistance is multifactorial, including obesity, physical inactivity, and dietary choices.

- Autoimmune Response: Type 1 diabetes is an autoimmune disease, where the immune system mistakenly targets and destroys insulin-producing cells in the pancreas.

- Obesity: Excess body weight, especially abdominal obesity, is a major risk factor for Type 2 diabetes. Fat cells release chemicals that can interfere with the body's ability to use insulin properly.

- Poor Diet: Consuming a diet high in refined sugars, unhealthy fats, and low in fiber can increase the risk of Type 2 diabetes. On the other hand, a balanced and nutritious diet can help prevent and manage the condition.

- Physical Inactivity: Sedentary lifestyles and a lack of regular exercise contribute to the development of Type 2 diabetes. Exercise helps the body use insulin more effectively and maintain healthy blood sugar levels.

- Gestational Factors: During pregnancy, hormonal changes can lead to gestational diabetes, particularly in women with risk factors such as obesity or a family history of diabetes.

Symptoms of Diabetes

While the symptoms of diabetes can vary depending on the type and the individual, there are some common signs to be aware of:

1. Increased Thirst (Polydipsia): People with diabetes often feel excessively thirsty due to increased urination and dehydration.

2. Frequent Urination (Polyuria): An excessive need to urinate is a common symptom. The body tries to eliminate excess glucose through urine.

3. Unexplained Weight Loss: Individuals with diabetes, especially Type 1, may experience sudden weight loss despite increased hunger. This is due to the body breaking down fat and muscle for energy when it can't use glucose effectively.

4. Extreme Hunger (Polyphagia): The body's cells are deprived of energy when there is not enough insulin or insulin is not working properly, leading to persistent hunger.

5. Fatigue: Diabetes can cause fatigue and a general sense of tiredness due to the body's inability to utilize glucose efficiently for energy.

6. Blurred Vision: High blood sugar levels can affect the lens of the eye, causing temporary blurriness.

7. Slow Wound Healing: People with diabetes may experience slow wound healing and are at an increased risk of infections.

8. Tingling and Numbness: This can occur in the hands and feet, a condition known as diabetic neuropathy.

It's important to note that some individuals may have diabetes and not experience any noticeable symptoms. Regular check-ups and blood sugar monitoring are essential, particularly for those with risk factors.

Diabetes is a pervasive condition with far-reaching implications for individuals and healthcare systems.

Understanding the types, causes, and symptoms is a crucial step in managing and preventing this chronic disease. With lifestyle modifications, early detection, and appropriate medical care, many people with diabetes can lead healthy and fulfilling lives. Education and awareness are key in the global effort to combat the diabetes epidemic, and ongoing research continues to provide hope for more effective treatments and eventual cures.

CHAPTER 2:

Achieving Optimum Health with a Diabetes Diet: Foods to Eat and Avoid

Diabetes is a chronic condition that necessitates careful dietary management to maintain optimum health. A well-balanced diabetes diet can help control blood sugar levels, prevent complications, and improve overall well-being. In this 500-word essay, we'll explore the foods to include and avoid in a diabetes diet to achieve optimum health.

Foods to Eat:

1. Complex Carbohydrates: Opt for complex carbohydrates that have a lower glycemic index, as they are digested more slowly, resulting in gradual blood sugar spikes. Whole grains like oats, quinoa, brown rice, and whole wheat products should be a staple in your diet.

2. Fiber-Rich Foods: Fiber aids in blood sugar control and promotes a feeling of fullness. Consume plenty of fruits, vegetables, legumes, and whole grains rich in fiber. This includes broccoli, carrots, lentils, and whole fruits.

3. Lean Proteins: Lean protein sources such as poultry, fish, tofu, and legumes are excellent choices. Protein helps stabilize blood sugar levels and provides essential nutrients for overall health.

4. Healthy Fats: Opt for sources of healthy fats like avocados, nuts, seeds, and olive oil. These fats are beneficial for heart health and can help improve insulin sensitivity.

5. Non-Starchy Vegetables: Leafy greens, tomatoes, peppers, and other non-starchy vegetables are low in carbohydrates and calories but high in vitamins and minerals. They are a valuable addition to your diet.

6. Low-Fat Dairy: Choose low-fat or fat-free dairy products like yogurt and milk for their calcium and protein content. These can be part of a balanced diet in moderation.

7. Nuts and Seeds: Small portions of unsalted nuts and seeds, such as almonds, walnuts, and chia seeds, can provide healthy fats and help control hunger.

8. Berries: Berries like blueberries, strawberries, and raspberries are low in sugar and high in antioxidants, making them a nutritious choice for a diabetes-friendly diet.

9. Fatty Fish: Fish rich in omega-3 fatty acids, such as salmon, mackerel, and sardines, are beneficial for heart health and can help reduce inflammation.

Foods to Avoid:

1. Sugary Beverages: High-sugar beverages like sodas, fruit juices, and sweetened iced tea can lead to rapid blood sugar spikes. These should be strictly limited or avoided.

2. Processed and Refined Grains: Refined grains like white bread, sugary cereals, and pastries lack fiber and can cause quick increases in blood sugar. Choose whole grains over their refined counterparts.

3. Sweets and Desserts: Cookies, cakes, candies, and other sugary treats should be occasional indulgences at most. They can wreak havoc on blood sugar levels.

4. Trans Fats: Trans fats found in many processed and fried foods are detrimental to heart health and can exacerbate insulin resistance. Check food labels for "partially hydrogenated oils" and avoid products containing them.

5. High-Sugar Condiments: Sauces and condiments like ketchup, BBQ sauce, and sweet dressings can hide a surprising amount of added sugar. Opt for alternatives with little or no added sugar.

6. Excessive Fruit Consumption: While fruits are generally healthy, some, like grapes and watermelon, have a higher sugar content. Limit portions of these fruits to manage blood sugar levels.

7. High-Sodium Foods: Foods high in sodium can lead to elevated blood pressure, which is a concern for individuals with diabetes. Reduce intake of processed and salty foods.

8. Alcohol: Alcohol can cause fluctuations in blood sugar levels. If you choose to consume alcohol, do so in moderation and monitor your blood sugar closely.

9. Starchy Vegetables: Vegetables like potatoes, corn, and peas are higher in carbohydrates. While they can be included in the diet, it's essential to be mindful of portions.

Achieving Optimum Health with Meal Planning:

In addition to understanding which foods to eat and avoid, effective meal planning plays a critical role in managing diabetes. Here are some key tips:

1. Portion Control: Pay attention to portion sizes to prevent overeating and help stabilize blood sugar levels.

2. Regular Meals: Stick to a regular eating schedule with balanced meals and snacks to avoid dramatic blood sugar fluctuations.

3. Carb Counting: Learn to count carbohydrates to better manage your blood sugar. Consult a dietitian for guidance.

4. Food Journal: Keeping a food journal can help you identify patterns and make necessary adjustments to your diet.

5. Blood Sugar Monitoring: Regularly monitor your blood sugar levels to understand how different foods affect you and make informed choices.

6. Consult a Dietitian: Working with a registered dietitian who specializes in diabetes can provide personalized guidance and support.

In conclusion, a diabetes diet should prioritize whole, nutrient-dense foods while limiting sugary and processed options. By following these guidelines, individuals with diabetes can better control their blood sugar, reduce the risk of complications, and improve their overall health. Achieving optimum health with diabetes is not only possible but within reach through informed dietary choices and lifestyle adjustments.

CHAPTER 3:

Core Benefits of Following a Diabetes Diet for Beginners

For individuals newly diagnosed with diabetes, embarking on a diabetes diet can be both a daunting and transformative experience. While it may require some adjustment and commitment, the core benefits of following a diabetes diet for beginners are significant and can lead to improved health, well-being, and diabetes management.

1. Blood Sugar Control:

One of the fundamental goals of a diabetes diet is to control blood sugar levels. A well-planned diet ensures that carbohydrates are managed effectively, preventing dangerous spikes and crashes in blood sugar. This control is crucial in preventing complications associated with diabetes.

2. Weight Management:

Many individuals with diabetes are either overweight or obese, and excess weight can exacerbate the condition. A diabetes diet helps with weight management by controlling

18

calorie intake and promoting a healthier body composition. Weight loss or maintenance can improve insulin sensitivity and overall health.

3. Reduced Risk of Complications:

Diabetes can lead to a range of complications such as heart disease, kidney problems, neuropathy, and vision issues. A well-balanced diet can reduce the risk of these complications by keeping blood sugar levels within a healthy range and promoting overall health.

4. Increased Energy Levels:

Stable blood sugar levels mean more consistent energy throughout the day. This prevents the fatigue and mood swings that can result from blood sugar fluctuations. Beginners on a diabetes diet often report feeling more energized and alert.

5. Improved Heart Health:

Heart disease is a major concern for individuals with diabetes. A diabetes diet typically focuses on heart-healthy choices, such as reducing saturated and trans fats, increasing fiber intake, and including heart-protective fats like those found in fish and nuts. This promotes better cardiovascular health.

6. Better Cholesterol Levels:

A diabetes diet emphasizes foods that can help lower LDL (bad) cholesterol levels and increase HDL (good) cholesterol. These changes can reduce the risk of atherosclerosis and related complications.

7. Controlled Blood Pressure:

High blood pressure often accompanies diabetes. A diabetes diet, which includes lower sodium intake and heart-healthy foods, can help regulate blood pressure, reducing the risk of stroke and heart disease.

8. Balanced Nutrition:

A well-structured diabetes diet ensures that individuals receive balanced nutrition with essential vitamins, minerals, and macronutrients. This is crucial for overall health and can help prevent nutrient deficiencies.

9. Enhanced Insulin Sensitivity:

A diabetes diet can improve the body's sensitivity to insulin, allowing it to use the hormone more effectively to control blood sugar. This can reduce the need for medication and insulin injections.

10. Support for Long-Term Lifestyle Changes:

Starting a diabetes diet as a beginner can serve as a foundation for long-term lifestyle changes. It encourages healthier eating habits, regular exercise, and an overall focus on wellness. These changes are essential for sustainable diabetes management.

11. Education and Empowerment:

A diabetes diet is a learning process. Beginners become more knowledgeable about their condition, how different foods affect their blood sugar, and how to make informed dietary choices. This knowledge empowers individuals to take control of their health.

12. Personalized Approach:

A diabetes diet can be tailored to individual needs and preferences. With the guidance of healthcare professionals, beginners can create a personalized plan that suits their lifestyle and dietary preferences.

13. Blood Sugar Testing and Awareness:

Following a diabetes diet often requires regular blood sugar monitoring. This practice increases awareness of the impact of different foods and meals on blood sugar levels, allowing individuals to make real-time adjustments to their diet.

14. Supportive Community:

Many people with diabetes find solace and encouragement by connecting with others who share their experiences. Engaging with support groups and online communities can provide emotional support and practical advice for those on a diabetes diet.

15. Prevention of Hypoglycemia:

A well-planned diabetes diet helps prevent episodes of hypoglycemia (low blood sugar), which can be dangerous. Beginners on a diabetes diet learn how to balance meals and snacks to avoid sudden drops in blood sugar.

In conclusion, a diabetes diet is not just a regimen; it's a path to better health, improved blood sugar control, and an enhanced quality of life. For beginners, the journey may seem challenging, but the core benefits of a diabetes diet far outweigh the initial adjustments. By embracing this dietary approach, individuals can take control of their diabetes, reduce the risk of complications, and pave the way for a healthier and more fulfilling future.

CHAPTER 4:

How to Follow a Diabetes Diet: A Comprehensive Guide

Following a diabetes diet is essential for managing blood sugar levels and overall health. For individuals diagnosed with diabetes, understanding and implementing a structured eating plan can be a critical step in achieving better control of their condition. This comprehensive guide provides insight into how to follow a diabetes diet effectively.

1. Seek Professional Guidance:

  - Before making any significant dietary changes, consult with a registered dietitian or a healthcare provider who specializes in diabetes care. They can help create a personalized plan tailored to your specific needs.

2. Understand Carbohydrate Counting:

  - Carbohydrates have the most significant impact on blood sugar levels. Learning to count carbohydrates is crucial. Know the carb content of common foods and learn to read food labels.

3. Portion Control:

- Managing portion sizes is essential. Be mindful of how much you eat, as even healthy foods can affect blood sugar when consumed in excess. Consider using measuring cups and a food scale to get a better idea of portion sizes.

4. Choose Whole Grains:

- Opt for whole grains like brown rice, quinoa, whole wheat pasta, and oats instead of refined grains. Whole grains contain more fiber, which helps stabilize blood sugar levels.

5. Monitor Fiber Intake:

- Fiber is beneficial for blood sugar control and overall health. Include high-fiber foods like fruits, vegetables, legumes, and whole grains in your meals.

6. Include Lean Proteins:

- Lean protein sources like skinless poultry, fish, tofu, and legumes can help stabilize blood sugar and provide essential nutrients.

7. Healthy Fats:

- Choose sources of healthy fats such as avocados, nuts, seeds, and olive oil. These fats are beneficial for heart health and can help improve insulin sensitivity.

8. Non-Starchy Vegetables:

- Non-starchy vegetables like leafy greens, tomatoes, cucumbers, and peppers are low in carbohydrates and calories but high in vitamins and minerals. They are a valuable addition to your diet.

9. Limit Sugary Foods and Beverages:

- Sweets, sugary snacks, and sugary beverages can lead to rapid blood sugar spikes. Limit or avoid these as much as possible.

10. Healthy Snacking:

- Plan nutritious snacks that won't disrupt blood sugar levels. Options include Greek yogurt, raw vegetables, unsalted nuts, and small portions of fruit.

11. Meal Timing:

- Establish regular meal and snack times to help regulate blood sugar levels. Consistency in meal timing can make it easier to manage diabetes.

12. Balanced Plates:

 - Create balanced meals by including a variety of foods. A general guideline is to fill half your plate with non-starchy vegetables, a quarter with lean protein, and a quarter with whole grains or other carbohydrates.

13. Monitor Blood Sugar:

 - Regularly check your blood sugar levels as directed by your healthcare provider. Monitoring helps you understand how your diet affects your blood sugar.

14. Adapt to Lifestyle Changes:

 - A diabetes diet is not just about what you eat; it also includes lifestyle changes. Incorporate regular physical activity into your routine and ensure you get enough sleep.

15. Hydration:

- Stay well-hydrated by drinking water throughout the day. Be mindful of sugary beverages, which can lead to blood sugar spikes.

16. Gradual Changes:

- It's essential to make dietary changes gradually. This can help you adjust to your new eating plan and reduce the risk of frustration or feeling overwhelmed.

17. Collaborate with a Support System:

- Share your diabetes management goals with friends and family. Their support can be invaluable in helping you stick to your diabetes diet.

18. Consistency:

- Consistency is key when following a diabetes diet. Over time, it becomes a natural part of your daily routine.

19. Stay Informed:

- Stay informed about the latest developments in diabetes management and dietary guidelines. Knowledge empowers you to make informed choices.

20. Practice Mindful Eating:

- Be mindful of your eating habits. Avoid distracted eating, and pay attention to hunger and fullness cues.

21. Seek Help and Support:

- Managing diabetes can be challenging. Don't hesitate to seek professional help and emotional support when needed. Support groups and diabetes educators can offer guidance and encouragement.

In conclusion, following a diabetes diet involves careful planning, portion control, and a focus on balanced, nutritious meals. A diabetes diet is not a one-size-fits-all approach, and it should be tailored to your specific needs and preferences. With the right knowledge, guidance, and commitment, individuals with diabetes can successfully manage their condition, achieve better blood sugar control, and improve their overall well-being. Remember, the journey to a healthier life with diabetes is a marathon, not a sprint, and every step counts towards a healthier you.

CHAPTER 5:

Complications of Diabetes Without Proper Diet Management

Diabetes is a chronic condition that requires careful management to prevent the development of complications. When individuals with diabetes do not adopt the right diet and maintain proper blood sugar control, the risk of various complications increases significantly. In this essay, we will explore the potential complications of diabetes when a proper diet is not adopted.

1. Cardiovascular Complications:

One of the most severe complications of unmanaged diabetes is the heightened risk of cardiovascular problems. High blood sugar levels can lead to the accumulation of fatty deposits in blood vessels, a condition known as atherosclerosis. This, in turn, can increase the risk of heart attacks and strokes. Individuals with uncontrolled diabetes are more likely to have high blood pressure and unhealthy cholesterol levels, further exacerbating their risk of heart disease.

2. Kidney Disease:

Diabetes is one of the leading causes of kidney disease. When blood sugar levels are consistently elevated, the kidneys are forced to work harder to filter waste products from the blood. Over time, this increased workload can lead to kidney damage, and in some cases, kidney failure. Kidney disease can ultimately necessitate dialysis or a kidney transplant.

3. Neuropathy:

Uncontrolled diabetes can damage the nerves throughout the body, a condition known as neuropathy. This can lead to symptoms such as tingling, numbness, and pain, particularly in the extremities. Foot problems are common among those with diabetes and can become serious, potentially leading to amputation if infections go untreated.

4. Eye Complications:

Diabetes can lead to a variety of eye problems, including diabetic retinopathy, cataracts, and glaucoma. Diabetic retinopathy is particularly concerning as it can result in vision loss and even blindness. Proper blood sugar control and regular eye check-ups are essential for managing and preventing these complications.

5. Skin Issues:

People with diabetes are prone to skin problems, especially when blood sugar levels are uncontrolled. Skin conditions such as bacterial and fungal infections, as well as slow wound healing, are common. Diabetic dermopathy, which causes brown patches on the skin, is another potential issue.

6. Hearing Loss:

Studies have suggested a link between diabetes and an increased risk of hearing loss. High blood sugar levels can damage the small blood vessels in the inner ear, which can lead to hearing impairment.

7. Increased Risk of Infections:

Elevated blood sugar levels can weaken the immune system's ability to fight off infections. People with diabetes are more susceptible to infections, including urinary tract infections, skin infections, and gum disease. Poor wound healing further compounds the risk of infection.

8. Foot Complications:

Diabetic foot problems can be particularly severe. High blood sugar can damage the nerves in the feet, leading to decreased sensation and making it difficult to notice injuries or infections. Left untreated, minor injuries can progress to severe ulcers or gangrene, often requiring amputation.

9. Alzheimer's Disease:

Research suggests a possible link between uncontrolled diabetes and an increased risk of Alzheimer's disease. The exact relationship is still being studied, but blood sugar imbalances and insulin resistance may contribute to cognitive decline.

10. Mental Health Issues:

Living with diabetes can be emotionally challenging, particularly when the condition is not well managed. The stress and emotional toll of dealing with a chronic condition can lead to mental health issues such as depression and anxiety.

11. Sexual Dysfunction:

Diabetes can impact sexual health, leading to issues such as erectile dysfunction in men and reduced sexual desire and satisfaction in both men and women.

12. Increased Mortality Risk:

Inadequate management of diabetes and its associated complications can ultimately increase the risk of premature death. Cardiovascular issues, kidney disease, and other complications can have life-threatening consequences.

In conclusion, diabetes is a complex condition that can lead to a myriad of complications if not properly managed, with cardiovascular problems, kidney disease, neuropathy, and eye complications being some of the most significant concerns. Proper blood sugar control through diet, medication, and lifestyle changes is essential for reducing the risk of these complications and maintaining a good quality of life. It's imperative for individuals with diabetes to work closely with healthcare professionals to develop a personalized management plan that includes a balanced diet, regular monitoring, and effective medication, if needed.

CHAPTER 6: BREAKFAST RECIPES

Here are 10 diabetes-friendly breakfast recipes with ingredients and preparation methods:

1. Greek Yogurt Parfait:

- Ingredients:

  - 1 cup of plain Greek yogurt

  - 1/4 cup of fresh berries (e.g., blueberries, strawberries)

  - 2 tablespoons of chopped nuts (e.g., almonds, walnuts)

  - 1 teaspoon of honey (optional)

- **Preparation:**

1. In a glass or bowl, layer the Greek yogurt, fresh berries, and chopped nuts.

2. Drizzle with honey if desired.

3. Enjoy a protein-packed, low-sugar breakfast.

2. Oatmeal with Cinnamon and Apples:

- **Ingredients:**

- 1/2 cup of rolled oats

- 1 cup of water or unsweetened almond milk

- 1/2 apple, diced

- 1/2 teaspoon of cinnamon

- 1 tablespoon of chopped walnuts (optional)

- Preparation:

1. Cook the oats with water or almond milk until they reach your desired consistency.

2. Top with diced apples, cinnamon, and chopped walnuts.

3. A warm, fiber-rich breakfast option to start your day.

3. *Veggie Omelette:*

- Ingredients:

- 2 large eggs

- 1/4 cup of diced bell peppers

- 1/4 cup of diced tomatoes

- 2 tablespoons of diced onions

- 1/4 cup of fresh spinach

- Salt and pepper to taste

- Preparation:

1. Whisk the eggs and season with salt and pepper.

2. Pour into a heated non-stick pan.

3. Add the diced vegetables.

4. Cook until set and fold the omelets in half.

5. A protein-packed, low-carb breakfast.

4. Chia Seed Pudding:

- Ingredients:

- 2 tablespoons of chia seeds

- 1 cup of unsweetened almond milk

- 1/4 teaspoon of vanilla extract

- 1/2 cup of fresh mixed berries

- Preparation:

1. Mix chia seeds, almond milk, and vanilla extract in a jar or bowl.

2. Refrigerate for at least 2 hours or overnight.

3. Top with mixed berries before serving.

4. A nutrient-rich, low-sugar pudding.

5. Whole Grain Toast with Avocado:

  - **Ingredients:**

   - 2 slices of whole-grain bread

   - 1/2 ripe avocado

   - A pinch of red pepper flakes

   - A sprinkle of black pepper

  - **Preparation:**

   1. Toast the whole-grain bread.

   2. Mash the avocado and spread it on the toast.

   3. Season with red pepper flakes and black pepper.

   4. A hearty, fiber-rich breakfast.

6. *Cottage Cheese and Fruit Bowl:*

- **Ingredients:**

  - 1/2 cup of low-fat cottage cheese

  - 1/2 cup of fresh mixed fruit (e.g., berries, melon)

  - 1 tablespoon of chopped nuts (e.g., pistachios)

- **Preparation:**

  1. Combine cottage cheese and mixed fruit in a bowl.

  2. Sprinkle with chopped nuts.

  3. A protein-packed, low-sugar breakfast option.

7. *Peanut Butter and Banana Smoothie:*

- **Ingredients:**

  - 1 ripe banana

  - 2 tablespoons of natural peanut butter

  - 1 cup of unsweetened almond milk

  - 1/2 cup of plain Greek yogurt

  - Ice cubes (optional)

- **Preparation:**

1. Blend all the ingredients until smooth.

2. Add ice cubes if desired.

3. A protein-rich, filling smoothie.

8. Scrambled Tofu with Spinach:

- **Ingredients:**

  - 1/2 cup of crumbled firm tofu

  - 1/2 cup of fresh spinach

  - 1/4 cup of diced bell peppers

  - 1/4 cup of diced onions

  - Turmeric and black salt to taste

- **Preparation:**

1. Sauté onions and bell peppers in a non-stick pan.

2. Add crumbled tofu and spinach.

3. Season with turmeric and black salt.

4. Cook until the tofu is heated through.

5. A protein-rich, low-carb option for a savory breakfast.

9. Cinnamon and Almond Baked Apple:

- Ingredients:

  - 1 apple, cored and halved

  - 1/2 teaspoon of cinnamon

  - 1 tablespoon of chopped almonds

  - 1 teaspoon of honey (optional)

- **Preparation:**

  1. Place apple halves on a baking sheet.

  2. Sprinkle with cinnamon and chopped almonds.

  3. Drizzlc with honey if desired.

  4. Bake until apples are tender.

  5. A warm, naturally sweet treat.

10. Smoked Salmon and Avocado Wrap:

- Ingredients:

- 1 whole-grain tortilla or wrap

- 2 ounces of smoked salmon

- 1/4 avocado, sliced

- 1 tablespoon of cream cheese (optional)

- Fresh dill or chives (optional)

- Preparation:

1. Lay out the whole-grain tortilla.

2. Spread cream cheese (if using) on the tortilla.

3. Layer with smoked salmon, avocado slices, and fresh herbs.

4. Roll up and enjoy a delicious, protein-rich wrap.

These 10 diabetes-friendly breakfast recipes offer a variety of options to kick-start your day while maintaining good blood sugar control. Remember to monitor your portion sizes, as individual dietary needs may vary. Always consult with a healthcare provider or a registered dietitian for personalized guidance in managing your diabetes through a balanced diet.

CHAPTER 8: LUNCH RECIPES

Here are 10 diabetes-friendly lunch recipes with ingredients and preparation methods:

1. Grilled Chicken and Quinoa Salad:

- **Ingredients:**

  - 4 oz boneless, skinless chicken breast

  - 1/2 cup cooked quinoa

  - 1 cup mixed greens

  - 1/4 cup cherry tomatoes

  - 2 tablespoons balsamic vinaigrette dressing (low-sugar)

- **Preparation:**

  1. Season the chicken breast with salt and pepper and grill until cooked.

  2. Slice the grilled chicken.

3. In a bowl, combine quinoa, mixed greens, cherry tomatoes, and grilled chicken.

4. Drizzle with balsamic vinaigrette.

2. Lentil and Vegetable Soup:

- Ingredients:

- 1/2 cup dry green or brown lentils

- 2 cups mixed vegetables (carrots, celery, onions)

- 4 cups low-sodium vegetable broth

- 1/2 teaspoon thyme

- Salt and pepper to taste

- Preparation:

1. Rinse lentils and add them to a pot with vegetable broth and vegetables.

2. Simmer until lentils are tender.

3. Season with thyme, salt, and pepper.

3. Tuna Salad Lettuce Wraps:

- Ingredients:

- 1 can (5 oz) of tuna, drained

- 2 tablespoons plain Greek yogurt

- 1/4 cup diced celery

- 1/4 cup diced red bell pepper

- Lettuce leaves for wrapping

- Preparation:

1. In a bowl, combine tuna, Greek yogurt, celery, and red bell pepper.

2. Spoon the mixture into lettuce leaves for a low-carb, high-protein wrap.

4. Quinoa and Black Bean Bowl:

- Ingredients:

- 1/2 cup cooked quinoa

- 1/2 cup black beans (canned, drained)

- 1/4 cup diced cucumber

- 1/4 cup diced red onion

- 2 tablespoons olive oil and lime juice dressing

- **Preparation:**

1. Combine quinoa, black beans, cucumber, and red onion in a bowl.

2. Drizzle with olive oil and lime juice dressing.

5. Grilled Veggie and Hummus Wrap:

- **Ingredients:**

- 1 whole-grain tortilla or wrap

- Assorted grilled vegetables (zucchini, eggplant, bell peppers)

- 2 tablespoons hummus

- Fresh spinach leaves

- **Preparation:**

1. Lay out the whole-grain tortilla.

2. Spread hummus over the tortilla.

3. Layer with grilled vegetables and fresh spinach.

4. Roll up and enjoy.

6. Chicken and Vegetable Stir-Fry:

- Ingredients:

- 4 oz chicken breast, sliced

- 2 cups mixed stir-fry vegetables

- 2 tablespoons low-sodium stir-fry sauce

- 1 cup cooked brown rice

- Preparation:

1. In a pan, stir-fry chicken until cooked.

2. Add mixed vegetables and stir-fry sauce.

3. Serve over brown rice for a balanced meal.

7. Spinach and Feta Stuffed Chicken Breast:

- Ingredients:

- 4 oz boneless, skinless chicken breast

- 1 cup fresh spinach

- 2 tablespoons crumbled feta cheese

- 1/2 teaspoon dried oregano

- Salt and pepper to taste

- Preparation:

1. Preheat the oven to 375°F.

2. Cut a pocket in the chicken breast and stuff with spinach and feta.

3. Season with oregano, salt, and pepper.

4. Bake until the chicken is cooked through.

8. Salmon and Asparagus:

- Ingredients:

- 4 oz salmon fillet

- 1 cup asparagus spears

- 1/2 lemon, sliced

- 1 tablespoon olive oil

- Fresh dill (optional)

- Preparation:

1. Preheat the oven to 400°F.

2. Place salmon and asparagus on a baking sheet.

3. Drizzle with olive oil, add lemon slices, and sprinkle with fresh dill if desired.

4. Bake until salmon is flaky and asparagus is tender.

9. Turkey and Avocado Lettuce Wrap:

- Ingredients:

- 4 oz turkey breast slices

- 1/4 avocado, sliced

- 1/4 cup diced tomatoes

- Lettuce leaves for wrapping

- Preparation:

1. Lay out lettuce leaves.

2. Layer with turkey, avocado, and tomatoes.

3. Roll up for a low-carb, high-protein wrap.

10. Egg and Vegetable Scramble:

- Ingredients:

- 2 large eggs

- 1/2 cup mixed vegetables (bell peppers, onions, spinach)

- 1 tablespoon olive oil

- Salt and pepper to taste

- Preparation:

1. Heat olive oil in a pan.

2. Add mixed vegetables and sauté until tender.

3. Whisk eggs and pour over the vegetables.

4. Cook until set, season with salt and pepper.

These 10 diabetes-friendly lunch recipes offer a range of options that prioritize balanced nutrition while managing blood sugar levels. As with any dietary plan, individual needs may vary, so it's essential to consult with a healthcare provider or a registered dietitian for personalized guidance in managing diabetes through a balanced diet.

CHAPTER 9: DINNER RECIPES

Here are 10 diabetes-friendly dinner recipes with ingredients and preparation methods:

1. Baked Salmon with Asparagus:

- Ingredients:

- 4 oz salmon fillet

- 1 cup asparagus spears

- 1 tablespoon olive oil

- 1/2 lemon, sliced

- Fresh dill (optional)

- Preparation:

1. Preheat the oven to 400°F.

2. Place salmon and asparagus on a baking sheet.

3. Drizzle with olive oil, add lemon slices, and sprinkle with fresh dill if desired.

4. Bake until the salmon is flaky and the asparagus is tender.

2. *Grilled Chicken and Vegetable Skewers:*

- **Ingredients:**

    - 4 oz boneless, skinless chicken breast, cut into cubes

    - Assorted vegetables (bell peppers, zucchini, cherry tomatoes)

    - Marinade (olive oil, garlic, herbs)

- **Preparation:**

    1. Marinate chicken in olive oil, garlic, and herbs.

    2. Thread chicken and vegetables onto skewers.

    3. Grill until the chicken is cooked through and vegetables are charred.

3. *Quinoa and Black Bean Stuffed Bell Peppers:*

- **Ingredients:**

    - 2 bell peppers

    - 1/2 cup cooked quinoa

    - 1/2 cup black beans (canned, drained)

- 1/4 cup diced tomatoes

- 1/4 cup diced onions

- 1/4 cup shredded low-fat cheese

- Preparation:

1. Cut the tops off the bell peppers and remove seeds.

2. In a bowl, combine quinoa, black beans, tomatoes, onions, and half of the shredded cheese.

3. Stuff the bell peppers with the quinoa mixture.

4. Top with the remaining cheese.

5. Bake until the peppers are tender.

4. Beef and Broccoli Stir-Fry:

- Ingredients:

- 4 oz lean beef slices

- 2 cups broccoli florets

- 2 tablespoons low-sodium stir-fry sauce

- 1 cup cooked brown rice

- Preparation:

1. In a pan, stir-fry beef until cooked.

2. Add broccoli and stir-fry sauce.

3. Serve over brown rice for a balanced meal.

5. Lemon Herb Grilled Shrimp:

- Ingredients:

- 4 oz shrimp, peeled and deveined

- 1 tablespoon olive oil

- Zest and juice of 1 lemon

- Fresh herbs (e.g., thyme, rosemary)

- Salt and pepper to taste

- Preparation:

1. In a bowl, combine olive oil, lemon zest, lemon juice, fresh herbs, salt, and pepper.

2. Marinate shrimp in the mixture.

3. Grill shrimp until they turn pink and are slightly charred.

6. Eggplant Parmesan:

- Ingredients:

- 1 small eggplant, sliced

- 1/2 cup whole wheat breadcrumbs

- 1/4 cup grated Parmesan cheese

- Marinara sauce (no added sugar)

- Preparation:

1. Dredge eggplant slices in whole wheat breadcrumbs mixed with Parmesan cheese.

2. Bake until eggplant is tender.

3. Serve with a side of marinara sauce.

7. Turkey and Vegetable Stir-Fry:

- Ingredients:

- 4 oz ground turkey

- 2 cups mixed stir-fry vegetables

- 2 tablespoons low-sodium stir-fry sauce

- 1 cup cooked quinoa

- **Preparation:**

1. In a pan, cook ground turkey until browned.

2. Add mixed vegetables and stir-fry sauce.

3. Serve over quinoa for a balanced meal.

8. Spaghetti Squash with Pesto and Cherry Tomatoes:

- **Ingredients:**

- 1 small spaghetti squash

- 2 tablespoons pesto sauce

- 1/2 cup cherry tomatoes, halved

- Fresh basil (optional)

- **Preparation:**

1. Cut the spaghetti squash in half, remove seeds, and bake until tender.

2. Scrape out the squash with a fork.

3. Toss with pesto sauce and cherry tomatoes.

4. Garnish with fresh basil if desired.

9. *Tofu and Vegetable Curry:*

- Ingredients:

- 4 oz firm tofu, cubed

- Mixed vegetables (e.g., bell peppers, snap peas, carrots)

- 2 tablespoons curry paste (low-sugar)

- 1 cup cooked brown rice

- Preparation:

1. In a pan, stir-fry tofu and mixed vegetables.

2. Add curry paste and simmer.

3. Serve over brown rice.

10. Cauliflower and Chickpea Bowl:

- **Ingredients:**

  - 1 cup roasted cauliflower florets

  - 1/2 cup cooked chickpeas

  - 1/4 cup diced cucumber

  - 1/4 cup diced red onion

  - 2 tablespoons tahini dressing

- **Preparation:**

1. In a bowl, combine roasted cauliflower, chickpeas, cucumber, and red onion.

2. Drizzle with tahini dressing.

These diabetes-friendly dinner recipes provide a variety of options for a balanced and nutritious evening meal. It's essential to consult with a healthcare provider or a registered dietitian for personalized guidance in managing diabetes through a balanced diet.

CHAPTER 10: SNACK AND DESSERT

Here are 4 diabetes-friendly snack and dessert recipes with ingredients and preparation methods:

1. Greek Yogurt and Berry Parfait (Snack):

- **Ingredients:**

  - 1/2 cup of plain Greek yogurt

  - 1/4 cup of fresh berries (e.g., blueberries, strawberries)

  - 1 tablespoon of chopped nuts (e.g., almonds, walnuts)

  - 1 teaspoon of honey (optional)

- **Preparation:**

1. In a glass or bowl, layer the Greek yogurt, fresh berries, and chopped nuts.

2. Drizzle with honey if desired.

3. Enjoy a protein-packed, low-sugar snack.

2. Dark Chocolate-Dipped Strawberries (Dessert):

- **Ingredients:**

  - Fresh strawberries

  - Dark chocolate (70% cocoa or higher)

- **Preparation:**

  1. Wash and dry the strawberries.

  2. Melt the dark chocolate in a microwave or on a stovetop with low heat.

  3. Dip each strawberry into the melted chocolate and let excess chocolate drip off.

  4. Place on a tray lined with parchment paper.

  5. Allow the chocolate to cool and harden.

  6. Enjoy a satisfying, lower-sugar dessert.

3. Apple Slices with Almond Butter (Snack):

- **Ingredients:**

  - Apple slices

- Almond butter (no added sugar)

- Preparation:

1. Slice an apple into wedges.

2. Dip the apple slices in almond butter.

3. A satisfying, fiber-rich snack that combines the natural sweetness of apples with healthy fats.

4. Chia Seed Pudding with Berries (Dessert):

- Ingredients:

- 2 tablespoons of chia seeds

- 1 cup of unsweetened almond milk

- 1/4 teaspoon of vanilla extract

- Fresh mixed berries

- Preparation:

1. Mix chia seeds, almond milk, and vanilla extract in a jar or bowl.

2. Refrigerate for at least 2 hours or overnight until the mixture thickens.

3. Top with fresh mixed berries before serving.

4. A nutrient-rich, low-sugar pudding for a guilt-free dessert.

These snack and dessert recipes are designed to satisfy your cravings while keeping blood sugar levels in check. Always be mindful of portion sizes and individual dietary needs, and consult with a healthcare provider or a registered dietitian for personalized guidance in managing diabetes through a balanced diet.

CONCLUSION

In the journey towards managing gout, this cookbook serves as a valuable resource, offering a comprehensive range of delicious recipes tailored to help individuals with gout enjoy flavorful meals while safeguarding their health. Gout, characterized by painful joint inflammation due to the accumulation of uric acid crystals, can be managed effectively through dietary adjustments. By embracing the principles of this cookbook, you are taking a significant step towards a life with reduced pain and improved well-being.

Our collection of recipes is designed with gout management in mind. These recipes prioritize ingredients that are low in purines, which are known to trigger gout attacks. They emphasize fresh vegetables, lean proteins, whole grains, and fruits to help lower uric acid levels and reduce inflammation. By following these recipes, you will not only reduce the risk of painful flare-ups but also enhance your overall health.

Remember that managing gout is not solely about what you eat but also about adopting a balanced lifestyle. Regular exercise, proper hydration, and adequate rest play essential roles in gout management. This cookbook serves as a compass, guiding you towards a healthier, more fulfilling life.

As you embark on this culinary journey, we offer you this special motivation: embrace the power of self-care. By making these dietary changes and taking charge of your health, you are showing love and care for yourself. Gout can be challenging, but with the right diet, you can gain control and enjoy life to the fullest. You deserve a life free from the grip of gout's pain, a life filled with vitality and joy. Each recipe within these pages is a testament to the possibility of living well with gout. So, go ahead, savor the flavors, cherish the meals, and embrace a future free from gout's grip. Your journey begins with every bite.

CONTACT US

Dear Reader,

If you have any questions, need further clarification, or require assistance with any aspect of the book, please do not hesitate to reach out to me. I am more than happy to provide additional insights, address your queries, or simply engage in a meaningful discussion.

Feel free to contact me at: IsabelleHartleyBooks@gmail.com. Your feedback and inquiries are always welcome.

FREE 60-DAYS MEAL PLANNER

FREE 30-Days Meal Planner, a priceless extra to get you started on the path to a more organized and healthy living. This meticulously curated planner is made to make meal planning easier, save you time, and help you meet your nutritional objectives. Having a month's worth of recipes makes it simpler than ever to stick to your diet goals. Prepare to enjoy the advantages of this wonderful resource!

DAILY MEAL PLANNER

Day: ....

BREAKFAST

____

____

LUNCH

____

____

DINNER

____

____

INGREDIENTS NEEDED

- ☐ _______________________________________
- ☐ _______________________________________
- ☐ _______________________________________
- ☐ _______________________________________

DAILY MEAL PLANNER

Day: ....

BREAKFAST

LUNCH

DINNER

INGREDIENTS NEEDED

DAILY MEAL PLANNER

Day:

BREAKFAST

LUNCH

DINNER

INGREDIENTS NEEDED

- [ ]
- [ ]
- [ ]
- [ ]

DAILY MEAL PLANNER

Day: ....

BREAKFAST

LUNCH

DINNER

INGREDIENTS NEEDED

- [ ]
- [ ]
- [ ]
- [ ]

DAILY MEAL PLANNER

Day:

BREAKFAST

____

____

LUNCH

____

____

DINNER

____

____

INGREDIENTS NEEDED

☐ ______________________________

☐ ______________________________

☐ ______________________________

☐ ______________________________

DAILY MEAL PLANNER

Day:

BREAKFAST

LUNCH

DINNER

INGREDIENTS NEEDED

DAILY MEAL PLANNER

Day:

BREAKFAST

LUNCH

DINNER

INGREDIENTS NEEDED

- [ ]
- [ ]
- [ ]
- [ ]

DAILY MEAL PLANNER

Day: ....

BREAKFAST

____

____

LUNCH

____

____

DINNER

____

____

INGREDIENTS NEEDED

☐ _______________________________________

☐ _______________________________________

☐ _______________________________________

☐ _______________________________________

DAILY MEAL PLANNER

Day:

BREAKFAST

LUNCH

DINNER

INGREDIENTS NEEDED

- [ ]
- [ ]
- [ ]
- [ ]

DAILY MEAL PLANNER

Day:

BREAKFAST

LUNCH

DINNER

INGREDIENTS NEEDED

- [ ]
- [ ]
- [ ]
- [ ]

DAILY MEAL PLANNER

Day:

BREAKFAST

LUNCH

DINNER

INGREDIENTS NEEDED

DAILY MEAL PLANNER

Day: ....

BREAKFAST

____

____

LUNCH

____

____

DINNER

____

____

INGREDIENTS NEEDED

☐ ____

☐ ____

☐ ____

☐ ____

DAILY MEAL PLANNER

Day:

BREAKFAST

LUNCH

DINNER

INGREDIENTS NEEDED

DAILY MEAL PLANNER

Day: ....

BREAKFAST

____

____

LUNCH

____

____

DINNER

____

____

INGREDIENTS NEEDED

☐ _____________________________________

☐ _____________________________________

☐ _____________________________________

☐ _____________________________________

DAILY MEAL PLANNER

Day: ....

BREAKFAST

____

____

LUNCH

____

____

DINNER

____

____

INGREDIENTS NEEDED

☐ _______________________________________

☐ _______________________________________

☐ _______________________________________

☐ _______________________________________

DAILY MEAL PLANNER

Day: ....

BREAKFAST

____

____

LUNCH

____

____

DINNER

____

____

INGREDIENTS NEEDED

☐ _______________________________

☐ _______________________________

☐ _______________________________

☐ _______________________________

DAILY MEAL PLANNER

Day:

BREAKFAST

LUNCH

DINNER

INGREDIENTS NEEDED

DAILY MEAL PLANNER

Day: ....

BREAKFAST

____

____

LUNCH

____

____

DINNER

____

____

INGREDIENTS NEEDED

☐ ___________________________________

☐ ___________________________________

☐ ___________________________________

☐ ___________________________________

DAILY MEAL PLANNER

Day:

BREAKFAST

LUNCH

DINNER

INGREDIENTS NEEDED

DAILY MEAL PLANNER

Day: ....

BREAKFAST

LUNCH

DINNER

INGREDIENTS NEEDED

- ☐
- ☐
- ☐
- ☐

DAILY MEAL PLANNER

Day:

BREAKFAST

LUNCH

DINNER

INGREDIENTS NEEDED

DAILY MEAL PLANNER

Day: ....

BREAKFAST

LUNCH

DINNER

INGREDIENTS NEEDED

DAILY MEAL PLANNER

Day: ....

BREAKFAST

____

____

LUNCH

____

____

DINNER

____

____

INGREDIENTS NEEDED

☐ _______________________________________

☐ _______________________________________

☐ _______________________________________

☐ _______________________________________

DAILY MEAL PLANNER

Day:

BREAKFAST

LUNCH

DINNER

INGREDIENTS NEEDED

- [ ]
- [ ]
- [ ]
- [ ]

DAILY MEAL PLANNER

Day:

BREAKFAST

LUNCH

DINNER

INGREDIENTS NEEDED

- [ ]
- [ ]
- [ ]
- [ ]

DAILY MEAL PLANNER

Day: ....

BREAKFAST

LUNCH

DINNER

INGREDIENTS NEEDED

- ☐
- ☐
- ☐
- ☐

DAILY MEAL PLANNER

Day: ....

BREAKFAST

____

____

LUNCH

____

____

DINNER

____

____

INGREDIENTS NEEDED

☐ ____________________________________

☐ ____________________________________

☐ ____________________________________

☐ ____________________________________

DAILY MEAL PLANNER

Day: ....

BREAKFAST

____

____

LUNCH

____

____

DINNER

____

____

INGREDIENTS NEEDED

☐ ____

☐ ____

☐ ____

☐ ____

DAILY MEAL PLANNER

Day: ....

BREAKFAST

LUNCH

DINNER

INGREDIENTS NEEDED

- [ ]
- [ ]
- [ ]
- [ ]

DAILY MEAL PLANNER

Day: ....

BREAKFAST

____

____

LUNCH

____

____

DINNER

____

____

INGREDIENTS NEEDED

☐ ____

☐ ____

☐ ____

☐ ____

DAILY MEAL PLANNER

Day:

BREAKFAST

LUNCH

DINNER

INGREDIENTS NEEDED

DAILY MEAL PLANNER

Day:

BREAKFAST

LUNCH

DINNER

INGREDIENTS NEEDED

- [ ]
- [ ]
- [ ]
- [ ]

DAILY MEAL PLANNER

Day: ....

BREAKFAST

____

____

LUNCH

____

____

DINNER

____

____

INGREDIENTS NEEDED

☐ ____

☐ ____

☐ ____

☐ ____

DAILY MEAL PLANNER

Day:

BREAKFAST

____

____

LUNCH

____

____

DINNER

____

____

INGREDIENTS NEEDED

☐ _______________________________

☐ _______________________________

☐ _______________________________

☐ _______________________________

DAILY MEAL PLANNER

Day:

BREAKFAST

____

____

LUNCH

____

____

DINNER

____

____

INGREDIENTS NEEDED

☐ ___________________________

☐ ___________________________

☐ ___________________________

☐ ___________________________

DAILY MEAL PLANNER

Day:

BREAKFAST

LUNCH

DINNER

INGREDIENTS NEEDED

- [ ]
- [ ]
- [ ]
- [ ]

DAILY MEAL PLANNER

Day:

BREAKFAST

LUNCH

DINNER

INGREDIENTS NEEDED

DAILY MEAL PLANNER

Day: ....

BREAKFAST

LUNCH

DINNER

INGREDIENTS NEEDED

DAILY MEAL PLANNER

Day: ....

BREAKFAST

____

____

LUNCH

____

____

DINNER

____

____

INGREDIENTS NEEDED

☐ _____________________________________

☐ _____________________________________

☐ _____________________________________

☐ _____________________________________

DAILY MEAL PLANNER

Day: ....

BREAKFAST

LUNCH

DINNER

INGREDIENTS NEEDED

- [ ]
- [ ]
- [ ]
- [ ]

DAILY MEAL PLANNER

Day:

BREAKFAST

LUNCH

DINNER

INGREDIENTS NEEDED

DAILY MEAL PLANNER

Day: ....

BREAKFAST

____

____

LUNCH

____

____

DINNER

____

____

INGREDIENTS NEEDED

☐ _____________________________________

☐ _____________________________________

☐ _____________________________________

☐ _____________________________________

DAILY MEAL PLANNER

Day: ....

BREAKFAST

____

____

LUNCH

____

____

DINNER

____

____

INGREDIENTS NEEDED

- [ ] ___________________________
- [ ] ___________________________
- [ ] ___________________________
- [ ] ___________________________

DAILY MEAL PLANNER

Day:

BREAKFAST

LUNCH

DINNER

INGREDIENTS NEEDED

DAILY MEAL PLANNER

Day:

BREAKFAST

____

____

LUNCH

____

____

DINNER

____

____

INGREDIENTS NEEDED

☐ _____________________________________

☐ _____________________________________

☐ _____________________________________

☐ _____________________________________

DAILY MEAL PLANNER

Day:

BREAKFAST

LUNCH

DINNER

INGREDIENTS NEEDED

- [ ]
- [ ]
- [ ]
- [ ]

DAILY MEAL PLANNER

Day:

BREAKFAST

____

____

LUNCH

____

____

DINNER

____

____

INGREDIENTS NEEDED

☐ _____________________________________

☐ _____________________________________

☐ _____________________________________

☐ _____________________________________

DAILY MEAL PLANNER

Day: ....

BREAKFAST

____

____

LUNCH

____

____

DINNER

____

____

INGREDIENTS NEEDED

☐ _______________________________________

☐ _______________________________________

☐ _______________________________________

☐ _______________________________________

DAILY MEAL PLANNER

Day:

BREAKFAST

LUNCH

DINNER

INGREDIENTS NEEDED

DAILY MEAL PLANNER

Day:

BREAKFAST

LUNCH

DINNER

INGREDIENTS NEEDED

DAILY MEAL PLANNER

Day:

BREAKFAST

____

____

LUNCH

____

____

DINNER

____

____

INGREDIENTS NEEDED

☐ _______________________________________

☐ _______________________________________

☐ _______________________________________

☐ _______________________________________

DAILY MEAL PLANNER

Day:

BREAKFAST

LUNCH

DINNER

INGREDIENTS NEEDED

DAILY MEAL PLANNER

Day:

BREAKFAST

LUNCH

DINNER

INGREDIENTS NEEDED

DAILY MEAL PLANNER

Day: ....

BREAKFAST

____

____

LUNCH

____

____

DINNER

____

____

INGREDIENTS NEEDED

☐ _____________________________________

☐ _____________________________________

☐ _____________________________________

☐ _____________________________________

DAILY MEAL PLANNER

Day: ....

BREAKFAST

____

____

LUNCH

____

____

DINNER

____

____

INGREDIENTS NEEDED

☐ _______________________________________

☐ _______________________________________

☐ _______________________________________

☐ _______________________________________

DAILY MEAL PLANNER

Day:

BREAKFAST

LUNCH

DINNER

INGREDIENTS NEEDED

DAILY MEAL PLANNER

Day:

BREAKFAST

____

____

LUNCH

____

____

DINNER

____

____

INGREDIENTS NEEDED

☐ _______________________________________

☐ _______________________________________

☐ _______________________________________

☐ _______________________________________

DAILY MEAL PLANNER

Day:

BREAKFAST

LUNCH

DINNER

INGREDIENTS NEEDED

DAILY MEAL PLANNER

Day:

BREAKFAST

____

____

LUNCH

____

____

DINNER

____

____

INGREDIENTS NEEDED

☐ _____________________________________

☐ _____________________________________

☐ _____________________________________

☐ _____________________________________

DAILY MEAL PLANNER

Day: ....

BREAKFAST

LUNCH

DINNER

INGREDIENTS NEEDED

- ☐
- ☐
- ☐
- ☐